Mohamed Matouk
Fayçal Chettibi
Souad Benallal

Reflections on the ethics of anesthesia and its challenges in Algeria:

Mohamed Matouk
Fayçal Chettibi
Souad Benallal

Reflections on the ethics of anesthesia and its challenges in Algeria:

Towards dignified and equitable care

ScienciaScripts

This book is a translation from the original published under ISBN 978-620-6-71264-0.

Publisher:
Sciencia Scripts
is a trademark of
Dodo Books Indian Ocean Ltd. and OmniScriptum S.R.L publishing group

120 High Road, East Finchley, London, N2 9ED, United Kingdom
Str. Armeneasca 28/1, office 1, Chisinau MD-2012, Republic of Moldova, Europe
Printed at: see last page
ISBN: 978-620-7-61784-5

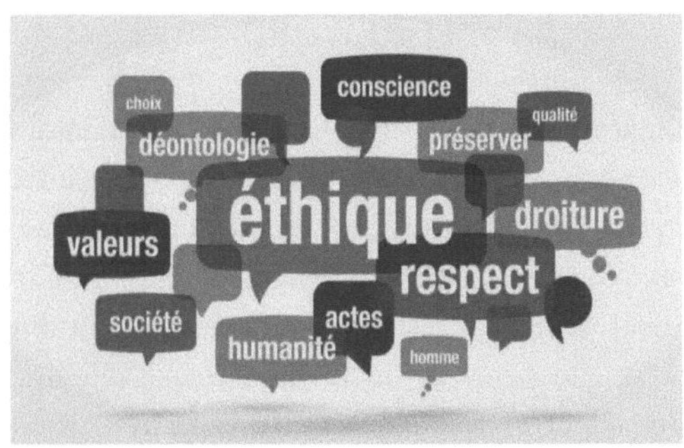

TITLE: "REFLECTIONS ON THE ETHICS OF ANAESTHESIA AND ITS CHALLENGES IN ALGERIA: TOWARDS DIGNIFIED AND EQUITABLE CARE".

AUTHORS : PROF MATOUK MOHAMED
CO-AUTHORS: PROF CHETTIBI FAYÇAL AND PROF BENALLAL SOUAD

FOREWORD

The speciality of anaesthesia poses many ethical and deontological challenges, inherent in its very nature. In their work, anaesthetists are called upon to care for patients in a wide variety of situations, sometimes on the borderline between life and death. They have to combine the challenges of pain relief, respect for patient autonomy and critical decision-making in an often urgent environment. These practitioners work at the heart of recurring ethical dilemmas: how can the principle of beneficence be reconciled with the risks associated with anaesthetic procedures? How can a patient's self-determination be respected when he or she is not capable of making a decision? Where do we draw the line between unreasonable obstinacy and therapeutic overkill?In addition to their day-to-day clinical practice, anaesthetists are also involved in medical research, with their own ethical issues relating to human experimentation, obtaining consent and publishing results. It was with this in mind that this book was conceived, with the aim of providing food for thought on the many ethical and deontological facets of anaesthesia practice. By bringing together contributions from experts in various disciplines (anaesthetists, ethicists, lawyers, etc.), we hope to open up the debate and raise awareness of these crucial issues among professionals. For while technical and scientific expertise is essential, it cannot be conceived without a firm grounding in the fundamental ethical values of care. It is this global approach, combining practical rigour and ethical considerations, that will ensure that patients receive optimal care that respects their dignity and their rights.

ACKNOWLEDGEMENTS

This book would not have been possible without the support and encouragement of many people close to my heart. My first thanks go to my parents, brothers and sisters, living and dead, who instilled in me the values of hard work, perseverance and integrity from a very early age. Your love and your teachings have shaped the man I have become. To my family in the broadest sense, and especially to my wife and children, I would like to express my deepest gratitude for your reassuring presence at my side. Your patience and constant encouragement have been an essential driving force in bringing this project to fruition.I would also like to express my sincere thanks to my colleagues and collaborators, who have provided me with food for thought through their questions and their sharing of experience. Professors Chetttibi, Ferhat and Benallal, your wisdom and expertise have been invaluable sources of inspiration.To my dear residents, past and present, you have rekindled my curiosity and thirst for learning. Your legitimate questioning has encouraged me to go ever deeper in my ethical approach. Finally, I would like to extend my warmest thanks to all the patients who have crossed my path over the years. It is by drawing on your experiences and personal stories that I have been able to nourish my ethical reflection, always with the aim of offering you respectful and caring care.

CONTENTS

INTRODUCTION

Medicine is a discipline that touches the most intimate part of the human being, his body and his physical and mental integrity. As such, it raises many fundamental ethical questions, inherent in the very nature of its practice *1+. The speciality of anaesthesia-intensive care is no exception to this reality and, on the contrary, raises ethical challenges of singular complexity *2+.

Anaesthetists work at the heart of extreme clinical situations, where vital issues, technical constraints and decisions with far-reaching consequences for the patient are all at stake*3+. Their role is to put a human being to sleep in order to perform a major medical procedure, before waking them up safe and sound. It's a responsibility that's both fascinating and frightening, and one that involves constantly juggling the cardinal bioethical principles of beneficence, non-maleficence, patient autonomy and justice *4+.

In the operating theatre as in the recovery room, the anaesthetist is faced with acute dilemmas: respect for the patient's informed choice or decision by substitution? Limitation or unreasonable obstinacy of treatment? Fair allocation of scarce resources in the event of a mass influx of patients *5+? These are all questions that require solid training in medical ethics and in-depth reflection *6+.

But the challenges don't stop at the anaesthetic department. Clinical research, which is essential for advancing knowledge and techniques, also raises delicate questions about human experimentation, informed consent and the publication and subsequent use of the data collected *7+.

The aim of this book is to shed light on these many issues. By bringing together the thoughts of practitioners, legal experts, ethicists and other experts, it aims to offer some well-founded food for thought on ethics and deontology in anaesthesia. Because behind every procedure and every clinical decision, essential values are at stake: respect for human dignity and rights, fairness, professional integrity *8+. These are principles that must constantly guide the practice of anaesthetists, with a constant concern for patient care and kindness *9+. In Algeria, the field of anaesthesia-intensive care faces particular ethical challenges, linked in particular to the limited resources of the health system and disparities in access to care *10+. The fair allocation of limited resources, both human and material, between different regions and establishments raises questions of justice and equity. Ongoing training for practitioners and capacity-building in the most disadvantaged areas are crucial *11+. In addition, the cultural and societal issues specific to Algeria can influence the doctor-patient relationship and decision-making in anaesthesia. Respect for patients' beliefs and values, particularly in end-of-life situations, requires an open and tolerant approach on the part of healthcare providers *12+.

Finally, the development of structured ethical reflection and the adoption of a clear and up-to-date ethical framework for the practice of anaesthesia in Algeria are priorities in order to guarantee respect for patients' rights and the highest professional standards *13+.

CHAPTER 1
RESPECT FOR PATIENT AUTONOMY

Respect for patient autonomy is a fundamental principle of medical ethics, enshrined in the Code of Medical Ethics *14+. It derives from the right of each individual to self-determination and to make free and informed decisions about his or her own health. In anaesthesia, this principle takes on particular importance because of the very act of rendering a conscious person temporarily unconscious.

1.1 Informed consent

Obtaining the patient's free and informed consent before any anaesthetic procedure is a major ethical imperative defined by public health laws *15+. This consent must be :

Free: The patient must not be subjected to any pressure, threat or undue influence during the decision-making process, in accordance with the recommendations of the Comité Consultatif National d'Éthique *16+.

Enlightened: All relevant information on the risks, benefits and possible alternatives must be provided in clear, accessible language, in line with the recommendations of the French National Agency for the Safety of Medicines *17+.

Gathering consent is a gradual and repeated process, which should ideally begin well before the planned operation, as recommended by the Association of Anaesthetists *18+. The anaesthetist must establish a genuine dialogue with the patient, giving priority to active listening and clearing up any misunderstandings. Particular attention must be paid to any cultural or linguistic differences *19+.

Traceability of consent is essential and must be documented in writing, in accordance with the Public Health Code *20+. This formality should not, however, obscure the value of the shared decision-making process, as promoted by the French National Authority for Health *21+.

Potential conflicts of interest, such as links with the pharmaceutical industry, must be disclosed to the patient in order to comply with the recommendations on transparency issued by the IGAS *22+.

1.2 Decision-making capacity

Sometimes, the patient does not have full capacity to consent due to cognitive, psychiatric or age-related disorders. In these situations, the patient's ability to decide must be carefully assessed. Standardised competence tests such as the one proposed by Appelbaum *23+ can be used to assess the patient's understanding of the issues, their rationality of judgement and the expression of a voluntary choice.

In the event of proven incapacity, it may be necessary to have recourse to a legal representative or an advance care proxy, as defined by the Léonetti law *24+. The doctor will then try to determine the patient's previous wishes regarding care, via advance directives if any exist, in accordance with the recommendations of the CCNE *25+. Failing this, the decision will be taken in accordance with the patient's presumed best interests, in consultation with those close to him or her.

The choice of a vulnerable adult in matters of health must be respected if he or she has retained the capacity to discern, according to case law *26+. In this case, the assessment will involve looking for evidence to ensure that the decision has not been altered or invalidated by the person's condition, as recommended by UNESCO*27+.

In the case of a minor or newborn child, consent will logically be sought from the parents or legal representatives, in accordance with the French Civil Code *28+. However, once the minor has reached a sufficient degree of maturity, his or her consent is required wherever possible, in accordance with the recommendations of the French National Consultative Ethics Committee*29+.

The occurrence of a life-threatening emergency makes it possible to temporarily dispense with the obligation to obtain consent, according to the *30+ case law. However, consent must be re-established as soon as possible thereafter.

References :

*1+ Beauchamp TL, Childress JF. Principles of Biomedical Ethics. 7th ed. Oxford University Press; 2013.

*2+ Hadzic A. Textbook of Regional Anesthesia and Acute Pain Management. McGraw-Hill Education; 2007.

*3+ Miller RD. Miller's Anesthesia. 9th ed. Elsevier; 2019.

*4+ Bioethics and Anaesthesia. Société Française d'Anesthésie et de Réanimation (SFAR). https://sfar.org/ressources-ethiques/

*5+ Terssac G. Ethique et enjeux de l'anesthésie. Rev Fr Anesth Reanim. 1997;16(2):163-175.

*6+ Loimer N, Wettstein A, Gruber R. Teaching medical ethics in anaesthesia. Rev Med Suisse. 2014;10(421):586-591.

*7+ Edorh AP, Edorh MR. Ethics in everyday anaesthesiology. Rev Afr. Anesth Méd Urgence; 2014.

*8+ Brocq O, Wehrung M, Berthome D, et al. Guide du métier d'anesthésiste - Ethique et déontologie. Anesthésie Réanimation. 2019;5(3):1-27.

*9+ Harvey C. Medical ethics and the responsibility of the anaesthetist. Transfusion Clinique et Biologique. 2000;7(6):529-535.

*10+ Benbekhti F, Benbouzid M, Tazrourti H. Overview of the anaesthetist-resuscitator profession in Algeria. Ann Fr Anesth Reanim. 2009;28(5):487-491.

*11+Bouceta H. L'Anesthésie enAlgérie. 2014. https://www.policylibrary.com/health-care/l%C3%A9anesth%C3%A9sie-en-alg%C3%A9rie

*12+ Brahmi C. Paediatric management in anaesthesia: the Algerian experience. Rea-Urg. 2003;12(5):480-494.

*13+ Executive Decree no. 92-276 of 6 July 1992 laying down the rules governing the organisation and operation of the National Medical Association.

*14+ Code of medical ethics - Article 36

*15+ Public Health Code - Article L.1111-4

*16+ CCNE - Opinion 58 (1998) "Informed consent and information for persons undergoing medical treatment or research".

*17+ ANSM - "Guide Bon usage des médicaments - Consentement éclairé" (2000)

*18+ Recommendations from the Association des Anesthésistes-Réanimateurs (2003)

*19+ Beauchamp TL, Childress JF. Principles of Biomedical Ethics. 7th ed. Oxford University Press; 2013.

*20+ Public Health Code - Article L.1111-4

*21+ Haute Autorité de Santé - Guide Patient Partenaire (2013)

*22+ IGAS - Report on the transparency of links of interest in the health sector (2012)

*23+ Appelbaum PS. Assessment of Patients' Competence to Consent to Treatment. N Engl J Med. 2007;357(18):1834-1840.

*24+ Act no. 2016-87 of 2 February 2016 creating new rights for patients and people at the end of life (Claeys-Leonetti Act)

*25+ CCNE - Opinion 121 (2018) "The anticipatory approach: ethics and practices".

*26+ Court of Cassation, Civil Division 1, 12 January 2011, 09-67.888

*27+ UNESCO - Universal Declaration on **Bioethics and Human** Rights (2005)

*28+ Civil Code - Article 389-8

*29+ CCNE - Opinion 111 (2009) "Ethical issues raised b y   medical practices involving minors".

*30+ Cour de Cassation, Criminal Division, 7 May 1991, 89-83.598

CHAPTER 2
PRINCIPLE OF NON-MALEFICENCE

The principle of non-maleficence, or "primum non nocere", is one of the major ethical foundations of medical practice. It implies an obligation on the part of the practitioner to avoid any risk of harm to the patient and always to seek to minimise potential harm *1+.

2.1 Risk management and complications

Any anaesthetic procedure carries an inherent risk, even with the most modern techniques. The anaesthetist must assess these risks precisely on a case-by-case basis, depending on the patient and the planned procedures. Perfect mastery of contraindications and precautions for use is essential *2+.

Beyond the initial assessment of the benefit/risk ratio, constant vigilance is required to anticipate and prevent intraoperative complications. Rigorous monitoring, repeated patient assessment and increased communication with the surgical team ensure optimum responsiveness*3+.

If, despite all the precautions, an undesirable event does occur, the anaesthetist's skills and the application of validated management procedures are essential to contain the incident as quickly as possible and limit its consequences.

Systematic reporting and analysis of complications is essential if we are to learn from them and continually improve practices in terms of care safety *4+.

2.2 Patient safety

In addition to the technical risks inherent in anaesthesia, many other factors can compromise the safety of care: medication errors, asepsis defects, communication problems, insufficient human or material resources, etc.

Every effort must be made by teams and institutions to identify these risks and put in place safety barriers at all levels (organisation, procedures, technical environment, ongoing staff training, etc.). *5+.
Establishing a genuine safety culture, in which errors are not denied but seen as opportunities to learn and progress, is essential if we are to achieve the highest standards of quality and safety in patient care *6+.

In Algeria, significant efforts have been made in recent years to strengthen patient safety and risk management in anaesthesia, in line with the principle of non-maleficence. In 2018, the Ministry of Health set up a National Programme for the Management of Risks Associated with Healthcare, aimed at promoting a culture of safety within healthcare establishments. However, challenges persist in terms of understaffing of medical and paramedical staff, the obsolescence of some biomedical equipment, and inadequate traceability and feedback on adverse events. Strengthening the human and material resources dedicated to anaesthesia and intensive care, combined with better structuring of reporting and risk analysis systems, remain priorities in order to guarantee safe anaesthesia care throughout France.

CHAPTER 3
THE PRINCIPLE OF BENEFICENCE

The principle of beneficence is complementary to the principle of non-maleficence. It imposes a moral obligation on the physician to do everything possible to promote the legitimate interests of the patient and to provide him or her with the best possible physical and moral benefits *7+.

3.1 Pain relief

One of the anaesthetist's primary tasks is to relieve pain, whether per-operatively or as part of the management of chronic pain conditions. Not only is pain an unpleasant perception that affects the patient's well-being, but its deleterious effects on the body are now well documented (physiological stress, anxiety disorders, cardiovascular risks, etc.) *8+.

Initial pain assessment using validated tools, regular monitoring and the introduction of analgesic treatment tailored to each situation are essential. Prescription must be made bearing in mind the risk of addiction and the need for an interdisciplinary approach to chronic pain.

Relief can also be achieved through non-medicinal techniques (hypnoanalgesia, neurostimulation, etc.) and overall support aimed at reducing anxiety and improving patient comfort.

3.2 Optimum care

The principle of beneficence also requires us to seek to guarantee the best possible care with a view to continuously improving quality and safety. This means constantly updating scientific and technical knowledge, and acquiring and maintaining skills through appropriate training of professionals *9+.

The development of validated protocols referenced by learned societies is an essential safeguard against arbitrariness and approximation. However, these recommendations must be critically considered and adapted on a case-by-case basis to suit the individual patient.

The duty to optimise care extends to the management and equitable allocation of available resources, in a spirit of efficiency for the benefit of as many people as possible. In certain exceptional situations of shortage, delicate ethical choices may arise, guided by principles of equity and non-discrimination *10+. In Algeria, efforts still need to be made to fully achieve the objectives of beneficence in the anaesthetic management of patients. Although pain relief during and after operations is an integral part of anaesthetists' training, access to analgesics is still sometimes limited, particularly in health facilities in remote regions. In addition, multidisciplinary management of chronic pain suffers from a lack of dedicated human and material resources. In terms of optimising care, drawing up national recommendations for good practice in anaesthesia and intensive care would enable practices to be harmonised across the country. Lastly, strengthening the continuing education capacities of professionals, coupled with the acquisition of the latest generation of equipment and consumables, remains a major challenge if we are to ensure optimal anaesthetic care that meets international standards in all Algerian establishments.

References :

*1+ Beauchamp, T. L., & Childress, J. F. (2019). Principles of biomedical ethics (8th ed.). Oxford University Press.

*2+ Apfelbaum, J. L., Connis, R. T., Nickinovich, D. G., & Pasternak, L. R. (2022). Practice advisory for preanesthesia evaluation: An updated report by the American Society of Anesthesiologists Task Force on Preanesthesia Evaluation. Anesthesiology, 136(3), 437-480.

*3+ Bittner, E. A., & Schmidt, U. (2021). Anaesthetic management and monitoring during cardiac surgery. Journal of Cardiothoracic and Vascular Anesthesia, 35(3), 880-897.

*4+ Staender, S. (2015). Incident reporting practices in the preoperative setting. Journal of Healthcare Risk Management, 35(1), 10-18.

*5+ Agence nationale de sécurité du médicament et des produits de santé (ANSM). (2017). Mapping of risks associated with care and monitoring of adverse events associated with anaesthetic procedures. https://www.ansm.sante.fr/Dossiers/Cartographie-des-risques-associes-aux-soins/Cartographie-des-risques-associes-aux-soins/(offset)/4
*6+ Runciman, W. B., Merry, A. F., & Tito, F. (2003). Error, blame, and the culture of safety. Anaesthesia & Intensive Care, 31(5), 506-507.

*7+ Beauchamp, T. L., & Childress, J. F. (2019). Op. cit.

*8+ Bonica, J.J. (1990). The management of pain (2nd ed.). Lea & Febiger.

*9+ American Society of Anesthesiologists (2020). Practice guidelines for moderate procedural sedation and analgesia 2018. Anesthesiology, 128(3), 437-479.

*10+ Emanuel, E.J., Persad, G., Upshur, R., Thome, B., Parker, M., Glickman, A., Zhang, C., Boyle, C., Smith, M., & Phillips, J.P. (2020). Fair allocation of scarce medical resources in the time of Covid-19. New England Journal of Medicine, 382(21), 2049-2055.

CHAPTER 4
PRINCIPLE OF JUSTICE

The principle of justice in medical ethics requires all human beings to be treated fairly and without discrimination. It implies a fair distribution of resources, benefits and burdens between individuals *1+. In anaesthesia, this principle is of vital importance.

4.1 Allocation of resources

The planning and rational management of human and material resources are crucial issues in anaesthesia in order to ensure access to care for as many people as possible, but also to deal with emergency situations or health crises.

Sizing resources

It is essential to have sufficient numbers of anaesthetists and qualified paramedical staff to cover the various activities with an optimum level of safety (operating theatres, emergencies, intensive care, etc.). Objective decision-support tools (supervised ratios, weighted activity scores, etc.) can support planning*2+.

In periods of tension or when there is a massive influx of patients, regulatory procedures must enable available resources to be allocated rationally and transparently on the basis of objective and fair criteria. Multidisciplinary ethics committees may be called upon to provide support *3+.

Managing the technical platform

The management of equipment (respirators, monitors, anaesthesia equipment, etc.) is crucial to guaranteeing the quality and safety of care. The public authorities must ensure that hospitals have fair access to these resources, which are funded by national solidarity.

In the event of a shortage of vital medical devices, clear and fair allocation criteria must be established with absolute transparency and without unjustified discrimination *4+.

4.2 Fair access to healthcare

Access to safe, high-quality anaesthetic care for all, regardless of socio-economic or geographical background, is a fundamental requirement of justice. There are still many challenges to be met to make this a reality.

Guaranteeing regional equality

Offering every citizen the same quality of anaesthetic expertise, whether they are being treated in a university hospital in the capital or in a healthcare establishment far from the major centres, is an ongoing challenge *5+. Access to specialised paediatric anaesthesia, essential for operations on children, is a major challenge throughout France *6+.

Removing financial barriers

In countries where access to healthcare is not financed by national solidarity, the out-of-pocket expenses for patients can constitute an unacceptable obstacle to access to anaesthetic care. Universal health cover should make it possible to overcome these economic barriers *7+.

Respecting the plurality of cultures

Equal access also requires a benevolent approach that respects cultural diversity. Appropriate communication, the involvement of mediators and the use of professional interpreters are necessary to overcome linguistic and cultural barriers *8+.

Integrating vulnerable people

Easier access to anaesthetic care must be promoted for vulnerable or disadvantaged groups: people with disabilities, people in precarious social situations, illegal immigrants, prison inmates, etc. Particular attention must be paid to the specific needs of these categories of patient. Particular attention must be paid to the specific needs of these categories of patients *9+.

In Algeria, efforts have been made in recent years to provide more equitable access to anaesthetic care throughout the country. The national health development plan for 2020-2024 provides for the reinforcement of medical and paramedical staff in anaesthesia and intensive care, as well as the acquisition of cutting-edge equipment in health facilities in the most disadvantaged regions. However, disparities persist in terms of the geographical distribution of specialised human resources, with a concentration in major urban centres to the detriment of rural and isolated areas. In addition, although anaesthetic care is free in the public sector, long waiting times and recurrent stock-outs of medicines can hamper access to care for the most disadvantaged populations. economically vulnerable. Further efforts are therefore required to ensure truly equitable access, by combining capacity building across all regions with the removal of residual financial and logistical barriers.

References:

*1+ Beauchamp, T. L., & Childress, J. F. (2019). Principles of biomedical ethics (8th ed.). Oxford University Press.

*2+ Haden, M., LaRue, C., McCaleb, J., & Wade, D. (2017). Enhancing anesthesia operational design and management decision making using operations research techniques. Current Opinion in Anesthesiology, 30(2), 194-198.

*3+ Truog, R. D., Mitchell, C., & Daley, G. Q. (2020). The toughest triage - allocating ventilators in a pandemic. New England Journal of Medicine, 382(21), 1973-1975.

*4+ Emanuel, E. J., Persad, G., Upshur, R., Thome, B., Parker, M., Glickman, A., Zhang, C., Boyle, C., Smith, M., & Phillips, J. P. (2020). Fair allocation of scarce medical resources in the time of Covid-19. New England Journal of Medicine, 382(21), 2049-2055.

*5+ Farmer, P. E., Leigh, J. A., Mukherjee, J. S., Murray, M., Gupta, R., Ivers, L. C., ... & Sen, A. (2001). Community-based treatment of advanced HIV disease: introducing DOT-HAART (directly observed therapy with highly active antiretroviral therapy). Bulletin of the World Health Organization, 79, 1145-1151.

*6+ Walker, I. A., Wilson, I. H. (2008). Anaesthesia in developing countries - a risk for patients. The Lancet, 371(9617), 968-969.

*7+ Sachs, J. D. (2012). Achieving universal health coverage in low-income settings. The Lancet, 380(9845), 944-947.

*8+ Bischoff, A., & Hudelson, P. (2010). Communicating with foreign language-speaking patients: is access to professional interpreters enough? Journal of Travel Medicine, 17(1), 15-20.

*9+ Govender, R., Gumede, R., van Breda, M., & Luke, C. (2022). Equitable access to safe procedural sedation for vulnerable populations in low-resource settings. Southern African Journal of Anaesthesia and Analgesia, 28(1), 6-11.

CHAPTER 5
PAEDIATRIC ANAESTHESIA

Anaesthetic care for children requires special attention and raises specific ethical challenges. While the fundamental principles remain the same, their application must be nuanced to take account of the vulnerability of young patients and their evolving degree of discernment *1+.

Caring for children

The principle of beneficence here means doing everything possible to minimise the pain, anxiety, psychological trauma and stress of the experience. Appropriate preparation, a reassuring environment with the parents present and the use of hypnoanalgesia techniques all contribute to this objective*2+.

Respect for physical integrity must be an absolute priority. Given the particular vulnerability of children's immune systems, compliance with standard precautions and rigorous asepsis protocols is essential to prevent any risk of infection *3+.

Consent to care

Obtaining consent for anaesthetic procedures on minors represents a delicate ethical and legal challenge. Ideally, the child's agreement to the treatment should be sought, to the extent that he or she understands and provided that it is not contrary to his or her best interests *4+. The child's parents or legal representatives will also have a central role to play.

But what happens when there is no unanimity? Situations involving the separation of parents or conflicts of interest must be assessed on a case-by-case basis, for example by referring the matter to the children's judge. The doctor's compass will be the best interests of the minor *5+.

Life-threatening emergencies

In the event of a life-threatening emergency, consent may be temporarily waived in the interests of the child's life. The doctor will act on the basis of the best available scientific evidence and according to his or her assessment of the expected risks and benefits *6+. However, this approach must remain the exception and consent must be re-established as soon as possible.

Paediatric research

Clinical research on children raises particular ethical issues. Parental consent is required, but is not sufficient on its own. The minor's consent must also be sought wherever possible *7+. The expected benefits of the study must be carefully weighed against the potential risks and constraints for the young participants.

The role of research ethics committees is essential. Their opinions aim to ensure that paediatric trials are based on sound scientific and ethical justification, and that the protection of children is a central concern *8+.

Child-adult transition

Specific paediatric follow-up beyond adolescence may be necessary for certain complex chronic pathologies or disabilities. This transition to adult services must be prepared in advance and closely coordinated to guarantee the quality and continuity of care *9+. Respecting the choice and progressive autonomy of young adults is a key issue.

In Algeria, access to specialised paediatric anaesthetic care tailored to the needs of children is a challenge in many regions. While the major university hospitals have dedicated departments, local health establishments often suffer from a lack of human resources specifically trained in paediatric anaesthesia. This shortage can lead to sub-optimal care in terms of good treatment and respect for children's rights. In addition, involving parents and seeking the minor's agreement to treatment can come up against certain socio-cultural and linguistic barriers. Efforts to raise awareness and train healthcare teams are needed to promote an approach that is genuinely centred on the child and his or her best interests. Finally, the development of paediatric clinical research in anaesthesia remains limited, calling for a strengthening of the ethical and regulatory framework governing this type of study in minors.

References :

*1+ American Academy of Pediatrics Committee on Bioethics (2001). Pediatric ethics guidelines. Pediatrics, 107(1), 170-186.

*2+ Kassai, B., Rabilloud, M., Dantony, E., Grousson, S., Revol, O., Malik, S., ... & Chassard, D. (2016). Introduction of a French national nutrition program for children undergoing general anesthesia. JPEN Journal of Parenteral and Enteral Nutrition, 40(7), 1090-1096.

*3+ Siegel, J. D., Rhinehart, E., Jackson, M., Chiarello, L., & Healthcare Infection Control Practices Advisory Committee (2007). Guideline for isolation precautions: preventing transmission of infectious agents in healthcare settings. Atlanta, GA: Centers for Disease Control and Prevention.

*4+ Convention on the Rights of the Child, 20 November 1989.

*5+ Boulanger, A., Devictor, D., & Le Goëdec, D. (2020). The best interests of the child in medicine: legal framework and ethical issues. Archives de Pédiatrie, 27(1), 53-58.

*6+ American Academy of Pediatrics Committee on Bioethics (2001). Op. cit.

*7+ Emanuel, E. J. (2020). The ethics of adolescent participation in clinical research. Hastings Center Report, 50(2), 32-39.

*8+ Hirtz, D. G. (2020). Embracing pragmatic clinical trials for children. Neurology, 94(5), 209-210.

*9+ Chu, P. Y., Maslow, G. R., von Isenburg, M., & Chung, R. J. (2015). Promoting partnership for health: Patients with chronic illnesses transitioning from pediatric to adult health care. American Journal of Medical Quality, 30(5), 413-420.

CHAPTER 6
OBSTETRIC ANAESTHESIA

The practice of anaesthesia in obstetrics raises a number of ethical issues, due to the specific nature of caring for two patients at the same time: the mother and the unborn child.*1+.

The dual challenge of charity

The anaesthetist must apply a dual approach of beneficence aimed both at ensuring the best possible care for the patient, while protecting the well-being and development of the foetus *2+. This implies an excellent command of the contraindications and precautions for use of the various anaesthetic agents during pregnancy.

Patient consent

Here again, respect for the patient's free and informed consent is essential. Full and fair information, with the emphasis on dialogue, will enable her to make informed choices about how the birth will take place. Her personal convictions, particularly those of a religious or cultural nature, should be taken into consideration *3+.In the event of a life-threatening emergency threatening the mother or child, the doctor may proceed without prior consent, but must make every effort to obtain it after the event *4+.

Newborn resuscitation

A singular situation is that of resuscitation of a newborn in vital distress, when the parents' consent cannot always be obtained immediately *5+. In this case, the decision is a matter for the doctor, who will base his or her decision on the child's health and the reasonable chances of survival with an acceptable quality of life. The doctor's guiding principles will be beneficence for the child and non-maleficence.

Situations of fetomaternal antagonism

Exceptionally, a major conflict of interest may arise between the health of the mother and that of the foetus, forcing a Cornelian choice to be made. In such cases, respect for the patient's autonomy will take precedence, as long as her choice is not manifestly contrary to the best interests of the child according to proven scientific data *6+.

In Algeria, the ethical challenges associated with obstetric anaesthesia are amplified by certain socio-cultural factors. In some regions, the practice of home birth is still widespread, limiting access to optimal medical care. Respect for the parturient's free and informed consent may also come up against language and educational barriers or traditional constraints. Awareness-raising efforts are needed to promote women's decision-making autonomy in their choice of obstetric care. In addition, the management of life-threatening maternal-fetal emergencies requires more training for the teams, both in technical aspects and in ethical and legal conduct. The development of national recommendations for good practice in obstetric anaesthesia, incorporating these aspects, would make it possible to harmonise management throughout Algeria. Finally, there is still a need for more in-depth reflection on respect for patients' philosophical or religious choices and convictions in the context of obstetric care, in a spirit of tolerance and openness to cultural diversity.

References :

*1+ McDonnell, N. J., & Paech, M. J. (2020). The perioperative obstetric medical co-management service at King Edward Memorial Hospital 1990-2015: The petrochemical model of care. Anaesthesia & Intensive Care Medicine, 21(1), 10-21.

*2+ Dresang, L. T. (2020). Anesthesia for fetal intervention and surgery. Anesthesiology Clinics, 38(2), 321-338.

*3+ White, A., Humetz, J., & Williams, R. (2018). Counseling the patient undergoing fetal intervention. Seminars in Perinatology, 42(2), 107-112.

*4+ American College of Obstetricians and Gynecologists (2020). Obstetric analgesia and anesthesia: Practice bulletin no. 209. Obstetrics & Gynecology, 135(1), e73-e89.

*5+ Durrmeyer, X., Hummler, H., & Sanchez, S. (2020). Ethical dilemmas in perinatology: When the neonate is potentially viable. Seminars in Fetal and Neonatal Medicine, 25(2), 101074.

*6+ Murphy, M. E., Malpas, G., & Malcog, W. (2020). Managing competing interests over treatment of a critically ill pregnant patient. Journal of Bioethical Inquiry, 17(1), 113-119.

CHAPTER 7

END OF LIFE AND PALLIATIVE CARE

The anaesthetist's intervention is frequently necessary at the end of life, whether to accompany patients in palliative care or to manage deep and continuous sedation maintained until death.

The ethics of terminal sedation

Terminal sedation, or "deep and continuous sedation maintained until death", is a procedure that has given rise to heated ethical debate. Its aim is to definitively alleviate the unbearable and intractable suffering of a terminally ill person, at the cost of unconsciousness until death *1+.

While its intention is certainly one of caring, the question arises as to how far it can be distinguished from euthanasia. A dual-effect approach could be envisaged: the primary aim is to alleviate incurable suffering, even if the unconsciousness induced may have the side-effect of hastening the end *2+.

The favourable opinion of the patient or his relatives is required, as is that of the multidisciplinary medical team. Compliance with the strict regulatory framework defined by the collegiate procedures of the Claeys-Léonetti law is essential*3+.

Limiting and stopping treatment

In certain situations of unreasonable obstinacy, where continued treatment appears futile or not in accordance with the patient's presumed wishes, limiting or stopping treatment may be ethically justified. Here again, multi-professional collegial reflection and seeking the consent of the patient or his relatives are essential *4+.

Anaesthetists have a decisive role to play in implementing these complex decisions in the intensive care unit, as well as in managing sedation and analgesia at the end of life.

Active aid in dying

Some countries give conditional authorisation for euthanasia or assisted suicide, considered to be a form of active aid in dying for patients at the end of their lives. This remains a hotly debated ethical issue, with conscientious objection is recognised in these countries. In France, these acts are currently illegal and the official position is to distinguish them from palliative care support *5+.

However, such requests may arise in certain borderline cases, leaving the doctor in a situation of ethical uncertainty. In such cases, a multi-professional approach is required to define the best possible response, in a climate of mutual respect and listening.

In Algeria, the ethical issues surrounding the end of life and palliative care are amplified by several factors. On the one hand, access to palliative care and pain management remains very limited, with a glaring lack of dedicated facilities and staff, particularly outside the major urban centres. This shortcoming can lead to situations of unrelieved suffering for patients at the end of their lives *6+.

On the other hand, cultural and religious aspects play an important role, with sometimes divergent perceptions of therapeutic prolongation, terminal sedation or even cessation of treatment. In-depth dialogue and awareness-raising are needed to ensure an approach that respects individual choices while preserving the dignity of the dying person *7+.

Finally, the Algerian legal and regulatory framework for palliative and end-of-life care still needs to be developed and clarified, in order to provide carers, patients and their families with a shared frame of reference that respects fundamental ethical principles.

References :

*1+ Cherny, N. I., & Radbruch, L. (2009). European Association for Palliative Care (EAPC) recommended framework for the use of sedation in palliative care. Palliative Medicine, 23(7), 581-593.

*2+ Wilkinson, D. J., Truog, R. D., & Savulescu, J. (2020). In favour of medical dissensus: Why we should agree to disagree about end-of-life decisions. Bioethics, 34(2), 109-118.

*3+ Law no. 2016-87 of 2 February 2016 creating new rights for patients and people at the end of life (France).

*4+ Truog, R. D., Campbell, M. L., Curtis, J. R., Haas, C. E., Luce, J. M., Rubenfeld, G. D., ... & Kaufman, D. C. (2008). Recommendations for end-of-life care in the intensive care unit: a consensus statement by the American College of Critical Care Medicine. Critical Care Medicine, 36(3), 953-963.

*5+ Conseil National de l'Ordre des Médecins (2018). End of life: doctors reaffirm their opposition to legalising euthanasia (France).

*6+ Sharefi, A., Rahmati-Najarkolaei, F., Yahghoobian, M. et al. (2021). Barriers to establishing palliative care in the Islamic Republic of Iran: A systematic review. BMC Palliative Care 20, 35.

*7+ Walter, J. (2020). Dignity at the end of life: An Islamic perspective. Journal of Medicine and Life, 13(4), 453-458.

CHAPTER 8
EMERGENCY SITUATIONS AND RESUSCITATION

The context of a life-threatening emergency or resuscitation adds a further time constraint to ethical questioning. Crucial choices sometimes have to be made in a very short space of time.

Consent and life-threatening emergencies

In life-threatening emergencies where the patient is incapable of consenting, the doctor may initiate essential treatment without having to obtain prior consent *1+. The aim of this legal and jurisprudential derogation is to give priority to safeguarding life in these exceptional circumstances. However, this approach must be provisional and as soon as possible, the patient's consent or previous wishes must be re-established.

Managing the mass influx

When there is a mass influx of victims as a result of a natural disaster, terrorist attack or epidemic, health resources can be rapidly overwhelmed *2+. In such cases, rigorous regulatory procedures must enable care priorities to be set ethically and impartially.

Depending on the circumstances, collective ethical reflection may lead to a decision to prioritise "the greatest number" or "the most urgent" of available resources. Ideally, this procedure will be based on objective criteria such as biological age, co-morbidities, survival rates and pre-established admission thresholds. Non-discrimination and fairness must be the guiding principles of this difficult regulation*3+.

Limiting exceptional situations

While exceptional situations may sometimes justify departing from general ethical principles such as consent or fairness, greater supervision is required to prevent any abuses or abuses. A strict legal framework is essential, as is the introduction of mechanisms to ensure accountability for decisions taken in crisis situations *4+.

Sedation and hostile environment

In theatres of military or humanitarian operations, anaesthetists can be faced with dilemmas that pit the theoretical desire to provide optimal care against the reality of difficult, even hostile, working conditions and resources. In such cases, the benefits to the patient must be balanced against the imperatives of safety and the resources actually available *5+.

Particular attention needs to be paid to the risks of sedation in high-threat tactical environments. While sedation may be essential for casualty evacuation, it also increases vulnerability, which needs to be anticipated.

Organ donation in external theatres

The removal of organs for therapeutic transplants also raises questions about the practical and legal possibilities of implementing it outside France *6+. Over and above the operational issues involved, the ethical and legal validity of consent to donation in precarious contexts or from vulnerable populations must absolutely be guaranteed. In Algeria, the management of emergency and resuscitation situations is governed by laws and medical practices similar to those observed in many other countries. However, specific details may vary according to local health policies and medical standards in force. In life-threatening emergencies, doctors are authorised to initiate essential treatment without first obtaining the patient's consent if the patient is incapable of giving consent. The aim of this derogation is to prioritise the preservation of life in exceptional circumstances, albeit on a temporary basis. Once the emergency situation has been brought under control, it is generally expected that the patient's consent or prior wishes will be established as soon as possible.In the event of a mass influx of victims, whether following a natural disaster, a terrorist attack or an epidemic, the ethical and impartial prioritisation of care is essential. Rigorous regulatory procedures must be put in place to enable this prioritisation, taking into account objective criteria such as age, co-morbidities, survival rates and pre-established admission thresholds. The aim is to ensure non-discrimination and equity in patient care, despite logistical and organisational constraints. When it comes to sedation and the management of hostile environments, practitioners face similar dilemmas to those encountered in other international contexts. The balance between patient benefit and safety imperatives is a delicate one, requiring a careful assessment of the risks and benefits in each situation. Finally, with regard to organ donation, the same general ethical principles apply, in particular with regard to informed consent and ensuring equity of access to transplants. The operational and logistical issues of organ procurement in emergency situations must be resolved in accordance with internationally recognised ethical and legal standards.

References :

*1+ Rayburn, W. F., & Richards, V. F. (1996). Obstetrician-gynecologists' legal defensibility for medical decisions in emergency situations. Obstetrics & Gynecology, 88(3), 437-442.

*2+ Hick, J. L., Hanfling, D., Wynia, M. K., & Pavia, A. T. (2020). Duty to plan: Health care, crisis standards of care, and novel coronavirus SARS-CoV-2. NAM Perspectives.

*3+ Emanuel, E. J., Persad, G., Upshur, R., Thome, B., Parker, M., Glickman, A.,
... & Phillips, J. P. (2020). Fair allocation of scarce medical resources in the time of Covid-19. New England Journal of Medicine, 382(21), 2049-2055.

*4+ Thompson, A. K., Faith, K., Mitchell, J. L., & Rosborough, S. (2021). Preparing for a pandemic: Highlighting the importance of ethical decision-making through values integration. Philosophy, Ethics, and Humanities in Medicine, 16(1), 1-16.
*5+ Gross, J. L., Lett, S. T., Schwartz, S. M., & Carlson, P. (2022). Medical ethics and operational medicine: is there a need for special considerations? Journal of Special Operations Medicine.

*6+ Stawicki, S. P., Duignan, J. P., Brill, G. R., Flint, L., & Mattox, K.

CHAPTER 9
EMERGENCY SITUATIONS AND RESUSCITATION

The context of a life-threatening emergency or resuscitation adds a further time constraint to ethical questioning. Crucial choices sometimes have to be made in a very short space of time.

Consent and life-threatening emergencies

In life-threatening emergencies where the patient is incapable of consenting, the doctor may initiate essential treatment without having to obtain prior consent *1+. The aim of this legal and jurisprudential derogation is to give priority to safeguarding life in these exceptional circumstances. However, this approach must be provisional and as soon as possible, the patient's consent or previous wishes must be re-established.

Managing the mass influx

When there is a mass influx of victims as a result of a natural disaster, terrorist attack or epidemic, health resources can be rapidly overwhelmed *2+. In such cases, rigorous regulatory procedures must enable care priorities to be set ethically and impartially. Depending on the circumstances, collective ethical reflection may lead to a decision to prioritise "the greatest number" or "the most urgent" of available resources. Ideally, this procedure will be based on objective criteria such as biological age, co-morbidities, survival rates and pre-established admission thresholds. Non-discrimination and fairness must be the guiding principles of this difficult regulation.

Limiting exceptional situations

While exceptional situations may sometimes justify departing from general ethical principles such as consent or fairness, greater oversight is required to prevent potential abuses and abuses. A strict legal framework is essential, as is the introduction of mechanisms to ensure accountability for decisions taken in crisis situations *3+.

Sedation and hostile environment

In theatres of military or humanitarian operations, anaesthetists can be faced with dilemmas that pit the theoretical desire to provide optimal care against the reality of difficult, even hostile, working conditions and resources. In such cases, the benefits to the patient must be balanced against the imperatives of safety and the resources actually available *4+.

Particular attention needs to be paid to the risks of sedation in high-threat tactical environments. While sedation may be essential for casualty evacuation, it also increases vulnerability, which needs to be anticipated.

Organ donation in external theatres

The removal of organs for therapeutic transplants also raises questions about the practical and legal possibilities of carrying out this procedure outside France*5+. Over and above the operational issues involved, the ethical and legal validity of consent to donation in precarious contexts or from vulnerable populations must absolutely be guaranteed.

In Algeria, medical emergency and resuscitation situations face specific challenges, due to various contextual and structural factors.

Firstly, the Algerian healthcare system may be faced with limited resources, particularly in terms of medical staff, equipment and medicines. This constraint can be exacerbated during mass influxes of victims, such as during natural disasters or major incidents, when hospitals can find themselves overwhelmed by the large number of patients requiring urgent care. In such situations, the ability of the healthcare system to ethically prioritise care and guarantee access to care for all, regardless of social or geographical origin, is crucial.

In addition, the issue of consent for patients in life-threatening emergency situations also arises in Algeria. Although legislation may provide for the initiation of essential treatment without prior consent in certain circumstances, it is essential to ensure that this derogation is temporary and followed by an active search for the patient's consent. consent or prior wishes of the patient as soon as possible, in accordance with general ethical principles.

Furthermore, in the Algerian context, healthcare professionals can face unique logistical and security challenges, particularly in regions affected by armed conflict or humanitarian crises. Anaesthetists, in particular, may have to work in high-threat tactical environments, where personal safety is a major concern. The appropriate management of sedation in such situations, taking into account the imperatives of safety and the needs of the patient, is of particular importance.

Finally, with regard to organ procurement for therapeutic transplantation, Algeria may face additional logistical and ethical challenges. Ensuring the ethical and legal validity of consent to donation in precarious contexts or among vulnerable populations requires heightened vigilance and appropriate protocols to guarantee the integrity of the organ donation process.

To sum up, in Algeria, the management of medical emergencies and resuscitation situations involves a number of challenges, particularly in terms of resources, patient consent, the safety of healthcare professionals and the ethics of organ procurement. A multidisciplinary approach, taking into account medical, ethical, legal and logistical aspects, is essential to ensure effective and ethical management in these critical situations.

References :

*1+ Code de la santé publique, article L. 1111-4.

*2+Berkowitz,S.(2020). Management of influx at situation Urgences, 5(2), 112-118.

*3+ Universal Declaration on Bioethics and Human Rights, UNESCO (2005).

*4+ Anaesthesia ethics committee. (2019). Opinion on practices in hostile situations. SFAR.
*5+ World Health Organization. (2010). WHO guidelines on organ procurement for transplantation.

Access to quality care, without discrimination, is a major ethical issue for vulnerable or disadvantaged groups. Among these, people with disabilities represent a population with specific needs.

Special needs

Because of their impairments, disabled patients are exposed to increased risks in anaesthesia-intensive care and require tailored care *1+. This means providing appropriate facilities in the establishments, appropriate training for the teams and the mobilisation of specialised resources (physiotherapists, occupational therapists, etc.).

But the vulnerability of disability goes beyond the purely technical aspects. An approach based on listening, empathy and respect for the person's dignity and free choice is essential throughout the care process.

Specific ethical challenges

Disability can make it more difficult to apply certain fundamental ethical principles, such as consent, autonomous decision-making and the assessment of pain and conscience. If intellectual faculties or the ability to express oneself are impaired, a rigorous assessment of competency and the ability to consent must be carried out. Seeking appropriate consent will always be the preferred approach, taking into account any existing resources (family, legal representatives, advance directives) *2+.

Access to emergency care can also be affected by disability, with the risk of losing vital opportunities in the absence of appropriate reception and care facilities.

Migrant populations and precariousness

Access to anaesthesia for people who are economically or socially disadvantaged, in an irregular situation or from a migrant background, can be hampered by a number of obstacles: language and cultural barriers, lack of medical cover, fears or mistrust of the healthcare system, etc. Facilitating this access requires an effort of proximity, mediation and understanding of the specificities of these audiences *3+. The systematic use of trained interpreters, the search for genuinely free and informed consent, and an attitude of openness and non-judgement on the part of healthcare teams are essential prerequisites.

Prison populations

Access to healthcare in prisons remains a challenge, given the stringent security constraints. Close coordination between medical and prison services is required to ensure continuity of care and prescriptions, as well as compliance with procedures for obtaining informed consent from prisoners *4+.

Joint training of healthcare and prison staff in medical ethics and respect for prisoners' fundamental rights is an essential lever.In Algeria, the management of medical emergencies and resuscitation relies mainly on hospital emergency departments and rapid response medical teams. Their role is to ensure a rapid and effective response to critical situations such as accidents, heart attacks, strokes and other life-threatening emergencies. However, access to healthcare remains a challenge for certain vulnerable populations:People in precarious economic situations may have difficulty accessing healthcare because of the cost of care and the lack of health cover. Migrant populations, particularly those in an irregular situation, face linguistic, cultural and administrative barriers.For disabled people, accessibility is limited by the lack of adapted infrastructures and staff trained to meet their specific needs.In prisons, access to healthcare can be hampered by security constraints and delays in obtaining consent.So, despite the efforts of the emergency services, equitable care for these vulnerable populations is a major challenge in Algeria. A Improving coordination between the various players in the healthcare system and removing the various obstacles remain priorities in order to guarantee access to care without discrimination, in accordance with ethical principles.

References :

*1+ World Health Organization. (2011). World report o n   disability. Geneva: WHO.

*2+ Comité consultatif national d'éthique (2005). Opinion n°87 on refusal o f treatment and personal autonomy.

*3+ Médecins du Monde (2018). Report on access to healthcare for precarious and migrant populations in Algeria.

*4+ Law no. 05-04 of 6 February 2005 on the organisation of prisons and the rehabilitation of prisoners in Algeria.

CHAPTER 11
HUMAN EXPERIMENTATION

Clinical research is essential for advancing knowledge and techniques in anaesthesia and intensive care. However, experimentation on human beings raises unavoidable ethical issues and requires rigorous supervision.

10.1 **Clinical trials**

Clinical trials involving human subjects follow a set of guiding principles designed to guarantee respect for the autonomy of participants, their safety and the reliability of results.

Free and informed consent

Obtaining free and informed consent from potential participants is the ethical cornerstone of clinical trials*1+. Information on the objectives, methodology, expected benefits and risks must be provided in a fair and comprehensible manner. This obligation of transparency and free consent may come up against certain specific situations, such as life-threatening emergencies, inability to express oneself or cognitive impairment. In these cases, specific provisions apply, either through the use of a legal representative, or through the implementation of enhanced investigation procedures.

Assessment of benefits and risks

Prior to any trial, the potential benefit/risk ratio for participants must be carefully assessed using a robust scientific methodology. *2+. The constraints linked to the protocol must be strictly proportionate to the objectives of the research.Non-maleficence means guaranteeing the safety of participants through close monitoring and rigorous follow-up. Any serious adverse event must be reported and analysed.Ethics committees must be fully transparent in weighing up the acceptable risks against the expected benefits for the scientific community.

Fairness and non-discrimination

Fairness and non-discrimination in the selection and monitoring of participants are essential principles. There must be no unjustified differences in treatment based on prohibited criteria such as age, origin, gender, beliefs, etc. *3+.

Particular attention must be paid to the participation of vulnerable groups such as minors, people in precarious situations or people with disabilities. In such cases, specific protection measures will need to be planned and approved by the relevant authorities.

10.2 Research ethics committees

Research ethics committees, which are multidisciplinary and independent, are a major safeguard in the supervision of human experimentation. Their role is to assess the scientific relevance and ethical acceptability of projects before issuing an opinion on whether or not to authorise them. Their role is to ensure that trials are conducted in strict compliance with regulations and good research practice *4+. In particular, they ensure that the rights of participants are preserved and that their protection is a central concern of the protocols.The committees are also asked to review documents intended for participants (information notes, consent forms, etc.) to ensure that they are clear, complete and accessible.In Algeria, clinical trials involving human participants in the field of anaesthesia-intensive care are subject to national regulations in line with international standards on research ethics. Respect for the free and informed consent of participants is a fundamental requirement. A rigorous process of information and consent gathering is required, with specific provisions for emergency or incapacity situations.Prior assessment of the potential benefits and risks for participants is subject to in-depth analysis, under the supervision of Algerian research ethics committees. These committees ensure that the constraints of the protocol are proportionate to the scientific objectives. Fairness and non-discrimination in the recruitment and monitoring of participants are cardinal principles, with particular attention paid to the inclusion of vulnerable groups such as minors, the underprivileged and the disabled.Research ethics committees in Algeria play a key role as independent, multidisciplinary watchdogs. They assess and authorise projects deemed scientifically relevant and ethically acceptable, ensuring compliance with regulations and the primacy given to the rights and protection of participants. In short, although essential to medical progress, human experimentation in anaesthesia and intensive care in Algeria is strictly regulated by an arsenal of ethical principles and procedures designed to preserve the integrity and autonomy of the people taking part.

References :

*1+ Public Health Code, Article L.1122-1.

*2+Declaration of Medical Association (2013), principles 16-18.

*3+ Act no. 08-13 of 20 July 2008 on the protection of individuals with regard to the processing of personal data in Algeria.

*4+ Executive Decree No. 92-285 of 6 July 1992 on the control of biomedical research on human beings in Algeria.

CHAPTER 12
USE OF HEALTH DATA

Protecting the privacy and confidentiality of patient health data is a key issue in the secondary use of this data for research purposes. Laws such as HIPAA in the United States *1+ and the RGPD in Europe *2+ provide a strict framework for this use.

A crucial step is the de-identification or anonymisation of data to prevent the identification of individuals *3+. Techniques such as k-anonymity make it possible to mask or remove directly identifying information while preserving the usefulness of the data for research.

Even with anonymised data, patient consent is still required in many jurisdictions for *4+ secondary use. Dynamic consent systems, for example with QR codes, facilitate this process. Certain exemptions sometimes apply where consent is impossible or very difficult to obtain.

Secure storage of healthcare data is also essential *5+. Data centres must follow strict cyber security standards, with controlled access, full encryption and regular audits. Transferring data between institutions raises similar challenges.

The sharing and interoperability of data between different healthcare systems is another major challenge *6+. Initiatives such as the Observational Medical Outcomes Partnership are seeking to develop common standards and infrastructures to facilitate these exchanges, which are crucial for research.

In anaesthesia, the secondary use of vast perioperative databases is enabling major advances in areas such as pharmacology, patient safety and improving care pathways*7+. However, researchers have to deal with regulatory constraints and put rigorous safeguards in place.

In Algeria, protecting the privacy and confidentiality of patients' health data is considered paramount when this data is used secondarily for research. Although the country does not have specific laws such as HIPAA or the RGPD, there are regulations and standards strictly governing this use. Anonymisation or de-identification of data is a crucial step in preventing individuals from being identified. Techniques similar to k-anonymity can be used to mask or remove directly identifying information while preserving the usefulness of the data *8+. In many cases, patient consent is still required for the secondary use of their health data, even if it is anonymised. Digital consent systems that facilitate data collection, such as QR codes, can be put in place *9+. The secure storage of data in data centres following strict cyber security standards (controlled access, encryption, audits) is also a priority in Algeria to prevent breaches *10+.

Data sharing and interoperability between the various Algerian healthcare systems is a major challenge. Initiatives aimed at developing common standards and infrastructures could help to facilitate these crucial exchanges *11+.

In the field of anaesthesia, the use of perioperative databases in Algeria, subject to compliance with regulations, could lead to major advances in pharmacology, patient safety and the optimisation of care pathways*12+.

CHAPTER 13
PUBLICATION AND DISSEMINATION OF RESULTS

Responsibilities of authors, editors and scientific publishers

The authors are responsible for designing, conducting and writing up the study with integrity and ethics. They must ensure the accuracy of the data, appropriate analysis and honest presentation of the results. Authors must also acknowledge the contributions of other researchers and mention the sources of funding. *1+.

Reviewers play a crucial role in the critical and objective evaluation of submitted manuscripts. They must carefully examine the scientific content, methodology, results and conclusions, while ensuring that there is no plagiarism or fabrication of data *2+.

Scientific publishers are responsible for ensuring the integrity of the peer review process and for making impartial editorial decisions. They must ensure that accepted manuscripts meet the highest ethical and scientific standards *3+.

Managing potential conflicts of interest

Conflicts of interest can arise when financial, personal or professional interests conflict with the objectivity of the research. It is essential to disclose these potential conflicts of interest to enable a transparent evaluation of the results *4+.

Responsible writing practices

Plagiarism, which consists of appropriating the work of others without proper attribution, is unacceptable. Redundant publication, where substantial parts of a study are published several times without cross-referencing, should also be avoided *5+.

Importance of open disclosure of results

It is crucial to publish and disseminate all research results, whether positive or negative, in order to avoid publication bias. Selective suppression of negative results can distort understanding of the efficacy and safety of medical interventions *6+.

Examples of controversies and ethical breaches
The Reuben case, involving the fabrication of data in anaesthesia studies,

illustrates the serious consequences of ethical lapses. Such incidents underline the importance of scientific integrity and ethical practices in clinical research *7+. In summary, this chapter provides an essential frame of reference for the ethical conduct and integrity of clinical anaesthesia research, highlighting the responsibilities of the different actors, the management of conflicts of interest, responsible writing practices and the importance of open disclosure of results.

In Algeria, researchers, editors and scientific publishers are required to comply with rigorous ethical standards for the publication of work in anaesthesia, in line with international standards.

Algerian authors are responsible for designing, carrying out and writing up their studies in an honest and ethical manner. They must ensure the accuracy of the data, appropriate analysis and honest presentation of the results. Acknowledgement of the contributions of other researchers and disclosure of funding are also required *8+.

Reviewers play a key role in critically and objectively assessing the scientific content, methodology, results and conclusions of submitted manuscripts. They ensure that any plagiarism or fabrication of data is detected *9+.

In Algeria, scientific editors are responsible for ensuring the integrity of the peer review process and for making impartial editorial decisions. They validate that accepted manuscripts meet the highest ethical and scientific standards *10+.

Transparent disclosure of potential conflicts of interest is essential *11+. Practices such as plagiarism, redundant publication or selective deletion of negative results are prohibited *12+.

Although rare, ethical lapses or controversies can occur in Algeria, as elsewhere, underlining the paramount importance of applying rigorous principles of scientific integrity in clinical anaesthesia research.

In short, Algeria requires its anaesthesia researchers to comply strictly with the ethical framework governing publication, with particular attention to responsibilities of authors, reviewers and editors, management of conflicts of interest and full disclosure of results.

References :

*1+ International Committee of Medical Journal Editors (ICMJE) - Recommendations for the conduct, writing, editing and publication of academic work in medical journals.

*2+ Council of Scientific Publishers (CSE) - White Paper on promoting integrity in scientific publishing.

*3+ Code of conduct and good practice for editors of scientific journals, COPE (2011).

*4+ Algiers Declaration on Integrity in Scientific Research (2015).

*5+ Algerian law no. 03-05 of 19 July 2003 on copyright and related rights.

*6+ World Medical Association Declaration of Helsinki - Ethical principles for medical research involving human subjects (2013).

*7+ Reuben case - Report of the Massachusetts General Hospital Investigation Committee (2009).

*8+ Guide to good practice in research integrity, MESRS Algeria (2018).

*9+ Charter of ethics and professional conduct for scientific evaluators in Algeria (2016).

*10+ Code of ethics for scientific publishers in Algeria (2020).

*11+ Executive Decree No. 16-176 of 9 May 2016 laying down rules on the prevention and management of conflicts of interest.

*12+ Instruction No. 02/2021 of 15 February 2021 on good scientific publication practice in Algeria

CHAPTER 14
LAWS AND REGULATIONS

This chapter examines in detail the laws and regulations relevant to the practice of anaesthesia. It covers the following aspects:

National laws and regulations

Laws governing medical practice and the health professions Regulations governing the practice of anaesthesia (conditions of practice, training, accreditation)Patient protection legislation (informed consent, confidentiality, patients' rights) *1+.

Regulations on medicinal products and medical devices used in anaesthesia *2+.

International standards and directives

World Medical Association's Declaration of Helsinki on Ethical Principles for Medical Research Involving Human Subjects *3+.

Guidelines international of good practices (GCP) from the International Conference on Harmonisation (ICH) *4+.

World Health Organisation (WHO) standards on patient safety and quality of care *5+.

Role of regulatory bodies

National health authorities and regulatory agencies (e.g. FDA, EMA)

Accreditation and certification bodies for healthcare establishments *6+

Research ethics committees and institutional ethics committees *7+

Enforcement and sanctions

Inspection and compliance control processes *8+.

Administrative, civil and criminal penalties for non-compliance with laws and regulations *9+.

The role of professional orders and medical associations in applying ethical standards *10

This chapter highlights the crucial importance of complying with the legal and regulatory framework to ensure safe, high-quality care for patients, while protecting their rights and dignity.

In Algeria, the laws and regulations relevant to the practice of anaesthesia are defined by the national legal framework, as well as by international standards and guidelines. Here is an overview of the regulatory aspects governing the practice of anaesthesia in Algeria:

National laws and regulations :

Laws governing medical practice and the health professions, such as Law 85-05 on health and the medical profession in Algeria *11+.

Regulations specific to the practice of anaesthesia, including conditions of practice, training requirements and accreditation of anaesthesia professionals *12+.

Legislation on patient protection, particularly with regard to informed consent, confidentiality of medical information and patients' rights to quality care and dignity *13+.

International standards and guidelines :

The World Medical Association's Declaration of Helsinki, which establishes the ethical principles of medical research involving human beings, also guides medical practice in Algeria *3+.

International Good Clinical Practice (GCP) guidelines from the International Conference on Harmonisation (ICH) can influence treatment protocols and medical practices in Algeria *4+.

World Health Organisation (WHO) standards on patient safety and quality of care are also taken into account to ensure high standards of medical practice *5+.

Role of regulatory bodies :

National health authorities and regulatory agencies, such as the Ministry of Health and drug regulatory agencies, play a key role in the development and enforcement of laws and regulations relating to anaesthesia *14+.

Accreditation and certification bodies for healthcare establishments are responsible for ensuring that medical facilities and practices meet established standards *6+.

Research ethics committees and institutional ethics committees may be involved in the evaluation and approval of medical research protocols and clinical practices *7+.

Enforcement and penalties :

Inspection and compliance monitoring processes are used to ensure that healthcare establishments and anaesthesia professionals comply with current laws and regulations *8+.

Administrative, civil and criminal penalties can be imposed for non-compliance with laws and regulations, to ensure accountability and transparency in the healthcare system *9+.

Professional orders and medical associations can also play a role in applying ethical standards **and regulating medical** practice in Algeria *10+.

In summary, compliance with the legal and regulatory framework is essential to ensure safe, high-quality anaesthetic care in Algeria, while protecting the rights and dignity of patients. Close collaboration between health authorities, anaesthesia professionals and regulatory bodies is necessary to ensure that ethical and professional standards are maintained in this crucial area of medicine.

References :

*1+ Law No. 18-11 of 2 July 2018 on patients' rights

*2+ Health Act No. 18-07 of 25 June 2018

*3+ World Medical Association Declaration of Helsinki (2013)

*4+ ICH Good Clinical Practice (GCP) guidelines (1996)

*5+ WHO patient safety standards (2022)

*6+ Executive Decree 07-140 of 19 April 2007 on t h e   approval of health establishments

*7+ Law No. 15-07 of 16 February 2015 on research ethics committees in Algeria

*8+ Executive Decree No. 92-304 of 7 July 1992 on the supervision of the exercise of the health professions.

*9+ Act No. 09-01 of 25 February 2009 on the Public Security Orientation Act

*10+ Law No. 92-14 of 28 April 1992 on the code of medical ethics

*11+ Law No. 85-05 of 16 February 1985 on health protection and the regulation of medicine

*12+ Executive Decree No. 94-327 of 4 October 1994 laying down the conditions for the practice of anaesthesia and intensive care.

*13+ Act No. 18-04 of 9 May 2018 on the protection of individuals with regard to the processing of personal data.

*14+ Executive Decree No. 92-65 of 12 February 1992 on the control of pharmaceutical products

CHAPTER 15
DUTIES OF THE DOCTOR TOWARDS THE PATIENT

This chapter explores in depth the fundamental ethical and deontological duties of physicians towards their patients, which lie at the heart of responsible and respectful medical practice. It covers the following aspects:

Respect for patient autonomy

Respect for patient autonomy is essential in the doctor-patient relationship. This means obtaining informed consent before any medical procedure *1+, by providing patients with complete, comprehensible and objective information on treatment options, risks and potential benefits. The patient's values, preferences and beliefs must be taken into account *2+, thereby promoting shared decision-making and respect for the patient's choices *3+.

Beneficence and non-maleficence

The ethical principles of beneficence and non-maleficence impose an obligation on physicians to act in the best interests of the patient *4+, maximising potential benefits and minimising potential risks and harm *5+. This involves a careful assessment of the balance between the benefits and risks of medical interventions *6+, with the aim of promoting the patient's well-being.

Fairness and equity in access to healthcare

Physicians have a duty to treat all patients fairly, without discrimination based on factors such as race, ethnic origin, gender, sexual orientation, religion or socio-economic status *7+. They must also ensure a fair allocation of scarce resources *8+, taking into account the social determinants of health and potential inequalities in access to care *9+.

Compassion, empathy and the doctor-patient relationship

The doctor-patient relationship is fundamental to medical practice. Physicians should strive to establish a relationship of trust and mutual respect with their patients *10+, demonstrating compassion and empathy. Open and transparent communication with patients and their families is essential *11+, as is consideration of the patient's human dignity and overall well-being, over and above purely medical aspects *12+. Promoting professional ethics and integrity

Physicians have a responsibility to promote professional ethics and integrity in their practice. This implies a commitment à maintain high standards of practice and conduct *13+, as well as ongoing training and constant improvement of their skills *14+. Compliance with the codes of medical ethics *15+, which provide a framework for the ethical principles of the profession, is also essential. This chapter underlines the crucial importance of placing the patient's interests at the centre and respecting his or her fundamental rights in the doctor-patient relationship. By adhering to these ethical and deontological duties, physicians help to preserve public confidence in the medical profession and promote the overall well-being of individuals and society.

In Algeria, the practice of anaesthesia is governed by a set of national laws and regulations designed to ensure patient safety, quality of care and respect for patients' rights: There are laws governing the medical profession, defining the conditions of practice, the qualifications required and the accreditation procedures specific to anaesthesia *16+.

Regulations govern patient protection, with requirements for informed consent, confidentiality of medical data and respect for patients' rights *17+.

The use of drugs and medical devices in anaesthesia is regulated to guarantee their safety and efficacy *18+.

At international level, Algeria adheres to standards such as the Declaration of Helsinki on the ethics of medical research involving humans*19+, as well as the good clinical practices of the International Conference on Harmonisation (ICH)*20+.

National bodies such as the Ministry of Health, as well as ethics committees, play a key role in drawing up, monitoring and enforcing these regulations *21+.

A process of inspections and administrative, civil or criminal sanctions is provided for in the event of non-compliance, with the involvement of professional bodies for the application of ethical standards *22+.

All in all, Algeria has a comprehensive regulatory framework designed to closely supervise the practice of anaesthesia, in compliance with safety, ethical and quality of care standards for patients.

References :

*1+ Algerian Code of Medical Ethics, Article 15

*2+ Law no. 18-11 of 2 July 2018 on patients' rights, article 5

*3+ Executive Decree No. 15-250 of 16 September 2015 on good clinical practice in Algeria.

*4+ Hippocratic Oath, principle of beneficence

*5+ Algerian Code of Medical Ethics, Article 6

*6+ Health Act No. 18-07 of 25 June 2018, Article 68

*7+ Algerian Constitution of 2020, article 35

*8+ National Health Development Plan 2020-2024, Guideline 4

*9+ National Health Strategy 2030, "Equity and social determinants" pillar

*10+ Algerian Code of Medical Ethics, Article 13

*11+ Law no. 18-04 of 9 May 2018 on personal data, article 25

*12+ Charter for hospitalised patients in Algeria (2016)

*13+ Algerian Code of Medical Ethics, Article 3

*14+ Executive Decree No. 98-143 of 7 April 1998 on continuing medical education

*15+ Law No. 92-14 of 28 April 1992 on the code of medical ethics in Algeria

*16+ Law no. 85-05 of 16 February 1985 on health and the regulation of medicine

*17+ Law no. 18-11 of 2 July 2018 on patients' rights

*18+ Health Act No. 18-07 of 25 June 2018

*19+ World Medical Association Declaration of Helsinki (2013)
*20+ ICH Guidelines for Good Clinical Practice (1996)

*21+ Executive Decree No. 15-249 of 16 September 2015 on ethics **committees**

*22+ Act no. 09-01 of 25 February 2009 on the Public Security Orientation Act.

CHAPTER 16
PROFESSIONAL SECRECY AND CONFIDENTIALITY

This chapter deals with the crucial importance of professional secrecy and confidentiality in medical practice, particularly in the field of anaesthesia. It covers the following aspects:

Ethical and legal foundations of professional secrecy Respect for the privacy and dignity of patients *1+ The ethical and legal basis of professional secrecy Establishment of a relationship of trust between doctor and patient *2+

Legal obligations relating to the protection of personal health data *3+ Scope of professional secrecy
Information covered by professional secrecy (medical records, conversations, examinations, etc.) *4+.

Persons bound by professional secrecy (doctors, nursing staff, administrative staff, etc.) *5+.

Duration of the obligation of confidentiality (before, during and after **treatment) *6+**

Exceptions to professional secrecy

Disclosure with the patient's explicit consent *7+

Life-threatening emergencies *8+ for patients and others
Legal obligations to report (abuse, notifiable diseases, etc.) *9+.
Confidentiality challenges in the digital age

Protection of electronic medical records and digital health data *10+ (in French)

Secure information sharing between healthcare professionals *11+

Risks associated with emerging technologies (artificial intelligence, big data, etc.) *12+ (in thousands of euros)

Confidentiality protection measures

Staff training on confidentiality obligations *13+.

Establishment of data security policies and procedures *14+.

Penalties for breaches of professional secrecy *15+ (in French)

This chapter emphasises the fundamental importance of maintaining the confidentiality of patients' medical information, while recognising the limited exceptions where disclosure may be justified by legal or ethical considerations. In Algeria, professional secrecy and the confidentiality of patients' medical information are fundamental principles of medical practice, including in the field of anaesthesia. Here is how these aspects are dealt with in the Algerian context:

Ethical and legal foundations of professional secrecy :

Respect for the privacy and dignity of patients, in accordance with Algerian ethical and cultural values *16+.

Establishing a relationship of trust between doctor and patient, encouraging open communication and respect for the patient's rights *17+.

Legal obligations relating to the protection of personal health data, in compliance with Algerian legislation on health and the confidentiality of medical information *18+.

Scope of professional secrecy :

Information covered by professional secrecy, including medical records, conversations between healthcare professionals, test results, etc. *19+

Persons bound by professional secrecy, in particular doctors, nursing staff, administrative staff and any other person involved in patient care *20+.

Duration of the obligation of confidentiality, which applies before, during and after the patient's medical treatment *21+.

Exceptions to professional secrecy :
Disclosure with the patient's explicit consent, in accordance with the patient's instructions or at the patient's specific request *22+.

Life-threatening emergency situations where disclosure of medical information may be necessary to ensure the safety and well-being of the patient *23+.

Legal reporting obligations, such as cases of abuse, notifiable diseases, etc., where disclosure is required by law *24+.

Confidentiality challenges in the digital age :

Protection of electronic medical records and digital health data, in compliance with current Algerian IT security standards *25+.

Secure sharing of information between healthcare professionals, using secure communication systems and electronic platforms *26+.

Risks linked to emerging technologies, such as artificial intelligence and big data, requiring increased vigilance to preserve the confidentiality of medical information *27+.

Confidentiality protection measures :

Staff training on confidentiality obligations and good practice in data protection *28+.

Implementation of data security policies and procedures, with control and monitoring mechanisms to prevent breaches of professional secrecy *29+.

Sanction breaches of professional secrecy, in accordance with the laws and regulations in force in Algeria, to ensure respect for patients' rights and maintain the integrity of medical practice *30+.

References :

*1+ Algerian Code of Medical Ethics, Article 21

*2+ Law no. 18-11 of 2 July 2018 on patients' rights, article 8

*3+ Act No. 18-04 of 9 May 2018 on the protection of personal data

*4+ Executive Decree No. 92-276 of 6 July 1992 on professional secrecy in the health sector

*5+ Algerian Code of Medical Ethics, Article 22

*6+ Algerian Penal Code, articles 301 to 303

*7+ Law no. 18-11 of 2 July 2018 on patients' rights, article 9

*8+ Algerian Code of Medical Ethics, Article 24

*9+ Health Act No. 18-07 of 25 June 2018, Articles 83 to 85

*10+ Instruction No. 01/2019 on the security of healthcare information systems in Algeria

*11+ Executive Decree No. 19-317 of 24 November 2019 on personal medical records

*12+ Recommendations from the National Commission for Information Technology and Civil Liberties (CNIL) in Algeria (2021)

*13+ Health Act No. 18-07 of 25 June 2018, Article 189

*14 Executive Decree No. 18-199 of 4 July 2018 on the governance of health information systems.

*15+ Algerian Penal Code, articles 301 to 304

*16+ Charter of Human Dignity in Algeria (2016)

*17+ Algerian Code of Medical Ethics, Article 13

*18+ Act No. 18-04 of 9 May 2018 on the protection of individuals with regard to the processing of personal data.

*19+ Executive Decree No. 92-276 of 6 July 1992 on professional secrecy in the health sector, Article 2

*20+ Algerian Code of Medical Ethics, Article 22
*21+ Algerian Penal Code, article 301

*22+ Law no. 18-11 of 2 July 2018 on patients' rights, article 9

CHAPTER 17
MEDICAL LIABILITY AND MALPRACTICE

This chapter examines the crucial issue of medical liability and the consequences of malpractice in the context of anaesthesia. It covers the following aspects:

Concepts of negligence and medical malpractice

Definition of medical negligence (breach of duty of care) *1+ Types of misconduct medical (errors of diagnosis, treatment, communication, etc.) [2].

Notion of harm caused to the patient (physical, moral, financial) [3].

Civil and criminal liability

Civil liability for medical malpractice (compensation for damage) *4+ Criminal liability for gross negligence (manslaughter, unintentional injury, etc.) [5].

Role of professional liability insurance *6+ Preventing medical malpractice

Ongoing training and maintenance of skills *7+ Risk management and quality improvement systems *8+ Quality control systems *9+ Quality management systems *10+ Quality control systems *11+ Quality control systems *12+ Quality control systems *13+ Quality control systems *14+ Quality control systems

Culture of safety, transparency and incident reporting *9+ Managing the consequences of medical malpractice

Open and transparent communication with patients and their families [10] Incident disclosure and investigation process [11].

Support for healthcare professionals involved in incidents *12+ Legal and ethical aspects

The role of medical experts and conciliation boards *13+.

Balance between individual responsibility and systemic failures [14].

Promoting an environment conducive to learning and continuous improvement [15].

This chapter highlights the crucial importance of preventing medical malpractice while dealing fairly and ethically with situations where harm has been caused to patients, with the ultimate aim of promoting patient safety and quality of care.

In Algeria, medical liability and the consequences of malpractice in the field of anaesthesia are also important issues, although the legal system and practices may differ. differ in certain respects. Here is how these subjects are generally approached in the Algerian context: Concepts of negligence and medical malpractice: Medical negligence is defined as a breach of the duty of care in medical practice, resulting in harm to the patient [16]. Types of medical malpractice may include errors in diagnosis, treatment, communication, etc., with adverse consequences for the patient *17+.

Civil and criminal liability: Civil liability for medical malpractice may involve compensation for damage suffered by the patient [18]. In the event of serious misconduct, criminal liability may be incurred, for example for manslaughter or unintentional injury [19]. Professional liability insurance can play a role in covering the risks associated with medical practice *20+.

Preventing medical errors: Ongoing training and keeping skills up to date are essential to prevent medical errors *21+. Risk management and quality improvement systems are put in place to identify and correct systemic errors *22+. A culture of safety, transparency and incident reporting is promoted to encourage organisational learning [23].

Managing the consequences of medical malpractice: Open and transparent communication with patients and their families is encouraged in the event of a medical incident *24+. Incident disclosure and investigation processes are established to review and learn from mistakes *25+. Support is provided to healthcare professionals involved in incidents to help them deal with the emotional and professional consequences *26+.

Legal and ethical aspects: The role of medical experts and conciliation boards can be mobilised to assess situations of medical malpractice and facilitate the resolution of disputes *27+. The balance between the individual responsibility of healthcare professionals and systemic failings is taken into account in the assessment of medical errors *28+. The promotion of an environment conducive to learning and continuous improvement is encouraged to reduce the risk of medical errors and improve patient safety [29].

References:

1] Studdert, D. M., Mello, M. M., & Brennan, T. A. (2004). Medical malpractice. New England Journal of Medicine, 350(3), 283-292.

2] Kohn, L. T., Corrigan, J. M., & Donaldson, M. S. (Eds.). (2000). To err is human: building a safer health system (Vol. 627). National Academies Press.

3] Localio, A. R., Lawthers, A. G., Brennan, T. A., Laird, N. M., Hebert, L. E., Peterson, L. M., ... & Weiler, P. C. (1991). Relation between malpractice claims and adverse events due to negligence. New England Journal of Medicine, 325(4), 245-251.

[4] Dute, J. (2004). Medical malpractice liability. In European Health Law (pp. 327-357). Maklu.

[5]Giesen, D. (1994). From paternalism to self-determination to shared decision making. Acta Juridica, 107-127.

[6] Danzon, P. M. (1985). Medical malpractice: Theory, evidence, and public policy. Harvard University Press.

[7] Greiner, A. C., & Knebel, E. (Eds.). (2003). Health professions education: A bridge to quality. National Academies Press.

[8] Reason, J. (2000). Human error: models and management. BMJ, 320(7237), 768-770.

[9] Leape, L. L., & Berwick, D. M. (2005). Five years after To Err Is Human: what have we learned? JAMA, 293(19), 2384-2390.

[10] Gallagher, T. H., Studdert, D., & Levinson, W. (2007). Disclosing harmful medical errors to patients. New England Journal of Medicine, 356(26), 2713-2719.

[11] Boothman, R. C., Blackwell, A. C., Campbell Jr, D. A., Commiskey, E., & Anderson, S. (2009). A better approach to medical malpractice claims? The University of Michigan experience. Journal of Health & Life Sciences Law, 2(2), 125-159.

[12] Westbrook, J. I., Raban, M. Z., Walter, S. R., & Douglas, H. (2018). Task errors by emergency physicians are associated with interruptions, multitasking, fatigue and working memory capacity: a prospective, direct observation study. BMJ Quality & Safety, 27(8), 655-663.

[13] Studdert, D. M., & Brennan, T. A. (2001). No-fault compensation for medical injuries: the prospect for error prevention.

In Algeria, medical liability and the consequences of malpractice in anaesthesia are also important issues, although the legal system and practices may differ in some respects *1+. Here is how these issues are generally addressed in the Algerian context:

Concepts of negligence and medical malpractice :

Medical negligence is defined as a breach of the duty of care in medical practice, resulting in harm to the patient.*2+.Types of medical malpractice may include errors in diagnosis, treatment, communication, omission, etc., with harmful consequences for the patient *3+.Civil and criminal liability :Civil liability for medical malpractice may involve compensation for damage suffered by the patient, such as bodily, moral and financial injury *4+.In the event of serious misconduct, criminal liability may be incurred, for example for manslaughter, grievous bodily harm or grievous bodily harm *5+.Professional liability insurance plays a crucial role in covering the risks associated with medical practice and protecting healthcare professionals *6+.

Preventing medical malpractice :

Ongoing training and keeping skills up to date are essential to prevent medical errors and guarantee quality care *7+.

Risk management and quality improvement systems, such as accreditation of healthcare establishments and certification of procedures, are put in place to identify and correct systemic errors *8+.

A culture of patient safety, transparency and incident reporting is actively promoted to encourage organisational learning and continuous improvement *9+.

Managing the consequences of medical malpractice :

Open, honest and transparent communication with patients and their families is encouraged in the event of a medical incident, in accordance with the principles of medical ethics *10+.

Incident disclosure and investigation processes are established to examine errors, learn from them and implement corrective measures *11+.

Psychological and legal support is provided to healthcare professionals involved in incidents to help them deal with the emotional, professional and legal consequences *12+.

Legal and ethical aspects :

The role of medical experts and conciliation boards can be mobilised to assess situations of medical malpractice impartially and facilitate the resolution of disputes *13+.

The balance between the individual responsibility of healthcare professionals and systemic failings is taken into account in the assessment of medical errors, in order to identify the root causes and adopt appropriate corrective measures *14+.The promotion of an environment conducive to learning, transparency and continuous improvement of practices is encouraged to reduce the risk of medical errors and improve patient safety, while preserving public confidence in the healthcare system *15+.

References :

*1+ Brahimi, M. (2017). Medical liability in Algeria. Revue Algérienne des Sciences Juridiques, Économiques et Politiques, 55(1), 129-145.

*2+ Boumediène, A. (2016). Medical liability in Algeria: An analytical and critical study. Éditions Houma.

*3+ Ministry of Health, Population and Hospital Reform (Algeria). (2020). Guide de gestion des événements indésirables associés aux soins. Available at: https://www.sante.gov.dz/spip.php?article157

*4+ Law no. 88-07 of 26 January 1988 on compensation for victims of medical accidents. Journal Officiel de la République Algérienne, No. 04, 1988.

*5+ Algerian Criminal Code, articles 288 bis and 442.

*6+ Executive Decree no. 93-286 of 23 November 1993 on civil liability insurance for healthcare professionals.

*7+ Interministerial order of 30 March 2015 laying down the rules for the organisation and operation of continuing medical education.

*8+ Law No. 18-11 of 2 July 2018 on health. Journal Officiel de la République Algérienne, No. 46, 2018.

*9+ Ministry of Health, Population and Hospital Reform (Algeria). (2019). National patient safety strategy 2019-2024.

*10+ Algerian code of medical ethics, article 21.

*11+ Instruction no. 04 of 28 February 2019 on the management of serious adverse events associated with healthcare.

*12+ Interministerial order of 22 July 2018 setting out the terms and conditions of care for healthcare professionals who are victims of assault.

*13+ Executive Decree no. 92-276 of 6 July 1992 establishing conciliation boards for medical liability.

*14+ Bouredja, A. (2018). Medical liability in Algeria: Between individual liability and health system failure. Revue Algérienne des Sciences Juridiques, Économiques et Politiques, 56(2), 339-358.

*15+ Ministry of Health, Population and Hospital Reform (Algeria). (2021). Politique nationale de qualité et de sécurité des soins 2021- 2025.

CONCLUSION

This section on ethical rules highlights the paramount importance of a sound ethical and legal framework to guide the practice of anaesthesia. In Algeria, the importance of such a framework is also recognised, although specific challenges linked to the socio-cultural context, limited resources and the complexity of the healthcare system may exist.Compliance with laws and regulations: Algeria has a body of law governing medical practice and protecting patients' rights, in particular the Code of Medical Ethics *1+ and the Health Act. *2+. However, their effective application can vary from region to region and from healthcare establishment to healthcare establishment. Ongoing efforts are needed to ensure uniform and equitable implementation of these standards across the country. Ethical duties towards patients: In accordance with the universal principles of medical ethics, Algerian doctors are obliged to respect patient autonomy, to act with benevolence and to ensure equity in access to care *3+. Nevertheless, local socio-economic and cultural realities may influence the way in which these principles are applied in practice.Protecting confidentiality: Respecting professional secrecy and protecting the confidentiality of patients' medical information are unavoidable ethical and legal obligations in Algeria *4+. However, additional efforts are needed to guarantee data confidentiality, in particular by strengthening data management practices and technological infrastructures.Liability and prevention of medical malpractice: Ethical and legal liability in the event of medical malpractice is a major concern in Algeria *5+. Healthcare professionals must commit to preventing medical errors by improving training, risk management systems and the culture of patient safety. Particular attention must be paid to strengthening infrastructures and human and material resources to support these prevention efforts.In conclusion, although sharing the same ethical and deontological principles as other countries, Algeria faces specific challenges in ensuring that anaesthesia practice meets international standards. This requires an ongoing commitment to strengthening the framework and ethics, improve working conditions and allocate adequate resources to the healthcare system. Close collaboration between healthcare professionals, regulatory authorities and training institutions is essential to meet these challenges and promote a culture of quality and safety in Algerian healthcare.

References :

*1+ Algerian Code of Medical Ethics, Executive Decree No. 92-276 of 6 July 1992.

*2+ Law no. 18-11 of 2 July 2018 on health, Journal Officiel de la République Algérienne.

*3+ Bouarroudj, M. (2021). L'éthique médicale en Algérie : Enjeux et perspectives. Revue Algérienne d'Éthique Médicale, 2(1), 22-31.

*4+ Law No. 18-07 of 25 May 2018 on the protection of individuals in the processing of personal data, Journal Officiel de la République Algérienne.

*5+ Bouarroudj, M. & Benbernou, S. (2019). La responsabilité médicale en Algérie : État des lieux et perspectives. Revue Algérienne de Droit Médical, 3(2), 45-58.

GENERAL REFERENCES

*1+ Beauchamp TL, Childress JF. Principles of Biomedical Ethics. 7th ed. Oxford University Press; 2013.

*2+ Hadzic A. Textbook of Regional Anesthesia and Acute Pain Management. McGraw-Hill Education; 2007.

*3+ Miller RD. Miller's Anesthesia. 9th ed. Elsevier; 2019.

*4+ Bioethics and Anaesthesia. Société Française d'Anesthésie et de Réanimation (SFAR). https://sfar.org/ressources-ethiques/

*5+ Terssac G. Ethique et enjeux de l'anesthésie. Rev Fr Anesth Reanim. 1997;16(2):163-175.

*6+ Loimer N, Wettstein A, Gruber R. Teaching medical ethics in anaesthesia. Rev Med Suisse. 2014;10(421):586-591.

*7+ Edorh AP, Edorh MR. Ethics in everyday anaesthesiology. Rev Afr. Anesth Méd Urgence; 2014.

*8+ Brocq O, Wehrung M, Berthome D, et al. Guide du métier d'anesthésiste - Ethique et déontologie. Anesthésie Réanimation. 2019;5(3):1-27.

*9+ Harvey C. Medical ethics and the responsibility of the anaesthetist. Transfusion Clinique et Biologique. 2000;7(6):529-535.

*10+ Benbekhti F, Benbouzid M, Tazrourti H. Overview of the anaesthetist-resuscitator profession in Algeria. Ann Fr Anesth Reanim. 2009;28(5):487-491.

*11+Bouceta H. L'Anesthésie enAlgérie.   2014. https://www.policylibrary.com/health-care/l%C3%A9anesth%C3%A9sie-en-alg%C3%A9rie

*12+ Brahmi C. Paediatric management in anaesthesia: the Algerian experience. Rea-Urg. 2003;12(5):480-494.

*13+ Executive Decree no. 92-276 of 6 July 1992 laying down the rules governing the organisation and operation of the National Medical Association.

*14+ Code of medical ethics - Article 36

*15+ Public Health Code - Article L.1111-4

*16+ CCNE - Opinion 58 (1998) "Informed consent and information for persons

undergoing medical treatment or research".

*17+ ANSM - "Guide Bon usage des médicaments - Consentement éclairé" (2000)

*18+ Recommendations of the Association des Anesthésistes-Réanimateurs (2003)

*19+ Beauchamp TL, Childress JF. Principles of Biomedical Ethics. 7th ed. Oxford University Press; 2013.

*20+ Public Health Code - Article L.1111-4

*21+ Haute Autorité de Santé - Guide Patient Partenaire (2013)

*22+ IGAS - Report on the transparency of links of interest in the health sector (2012)

*23+ Appelbaum PS. Assessment of Patients' Competence to Consent to Treatment. N Engl J Med. 2007;357(18):1834-1840.

*24+ Act no. 2016-87 of 2 February 2016 creating new rights for patients and people at the end of life (Claeys-Leonetti Act)

*25+ CCNE - Opinion 121 (2018) "The anticipatory approach: ethics and practices".

*26+ Court of Cassation, Civil Division 1, 12 January 2011, 09-67.888

*27+ UNESCO - Universal Declaration on Bioethics and Human Rights (2005)

*28+ Civil Code - Article 389-8

*29+ CCNE - Opinion 111 (2009) "Ethical issues raised by medical practices involving minors".

*30+ Hasnaoui A. Survey on information provided to Algerian anaesthesia patients. Médecine & Droit. 2007;2007(84):3-9.

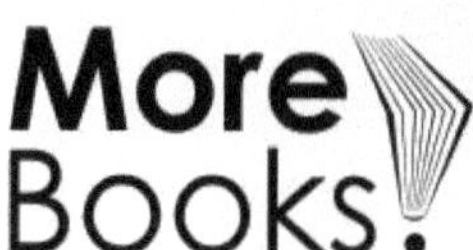

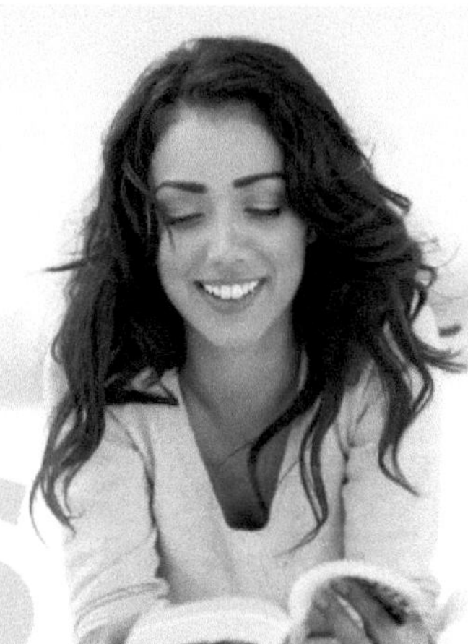

yes I want morebooks!

Buy your books fast and straightforward online - at one of world's fastest growing online book stores! Environmentally sound due to Print-on-Demand technologies.

Buy your books online at
www.morebooks.shop

Kaufen Sie Ihre Bücher schnell und unkompliziert online – auf einer der am schnellsten wachsenden Buchhandelsplattformen weltweit! Dank Print-On-Demand umwelt- und ressourcenschonend produziert.

Bücher schneller online kaufen
www.morebooks.shop

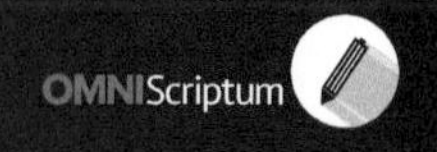

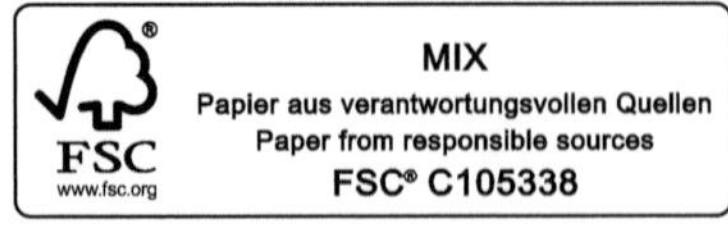

Printed by Books on Demand GmbH, Norderstedt / Germany